S.E.C.R.E.T.S!
21- DAY DEVOTIONAL

(Spiritually Equipping Christians Regarding Eating To Survive)

Spiritual Nourishment in the Word of God.

SECRETS!

Table of Content

INTRODUCTION

Have you ever heard that the Bible is meant to be food for Christians? Yet many of us frequently experience feeling spiritually dry, thirsty, hungry and even empty deep inside. We can even experience these feelings right after we have finished reading or studying the Bible. Why is that? In our reading and studying the Bible, we might learn something new, pick up some good advice or receive some inspiration, but it does not satisfy us. Despite our studying, we still feel hungry inwardly and we continue to feel that we are not just spiritually weak but spiritually dead. We know, of course, that books are meant to be read. If the book is a textbook for class, we read it, study it, and possibly commit some of it to memory. Or we might read the biography of a renowned person for inspiration and encouragement. But what about the Bible? Is it a book we read simply for inspiration or a textbook for us to learn about God and the Christian faith? Is it a book that instructs us how to be a good person or how to have a happy life? As Christians, we certainly should read God's Word regularly and even study it. But the Bible is not simply a work of literature, a textbook, or a self-help book. God's aim in giving His written Word to us was not that we would learn more doctrines, ethics and how to or even that we only be inspired. It was that we be Fed. Our lives consist of many matters, but the foremost matter for our physical survival is food. Only eating food satisfies our hunger and nourishes us. Without eating, we simply cannot continue to exist. In the same way, in order for believers to be healthy and grow in the divine life is to eat spiritual food. But what is the food for our spiritual life? God gave His Word to us to be our spiritual food. So even more than studying the Bible, we actually need to "eat" it. Nothing is more important to our Christian life than our being nourished with the Word of God. Biblical knowledge cannot help us if we are spiritually famished and consequently weak and dying. God's primary concern for us is that we would be living and growing by eating the Word of God as our food.

In this book the SECRETS, you will be equipped with nutrients from the Word of God which will help you to survive spiritually.

DAY 1: Are you thirsty for Jesus?

Scripture: **Psalms 63vs1 O God, you are my God. I earnestly search for you. My soul thirsts for you; my whole body longs for you.**

What does it look like to thirst for God? I have used that phrase in prayer that is hunger and thirst for God. What does that mean? Another powerful line is "My whole body longs for you in this parched and weary land." These are both beautiful imagery phrases which simply means that we must truly rely and rest in God no matter the circumstances and especially when we are weak and lonely. Are you living in desolation, feeling cut off from God and insecure about your future? Sometimes we do not even realize how parched we are. We keep filling our days with other things to fill the emptiness. We need to realize the weariness is a life devoid of relationship with our Creator. We are orphans searching for meaning. We can say "I know God" or "I'm a follower," but words are just words. Are we thirsting? Truly thirsting and hungry for more of a relationship? Maybe we do not have a relationship yet, but do recognize the emptiness. That is your yearning for God. Imagine seeing God present in your home. What is your response? In awe? In denial? Do you fall down on your knees? Are you overflowing with devotion and joy that the praises inside cries out?

Prayer: **Lord, draw me closer to you. I want to be where you want me to be and who you want me to become. I am feeling overwhelmed with balancing the desire to stay where it is safe and to go out and change the world, spreading your love one person at a time. Lord, I love you and I am seeking your direction. I am thirsty in this barren land. Fill me up. I am listening to your voice. In Jesus name. Amen.**

DAY 2: Abide in Jesus

<u>Scripture</u>: John 15 vs 4-5 "Abide in Me, and I in you. As the branch cannot bear fruit of itself unless it abides in the vine, no neither can you unless you abide in Me, I am the vine, you are the branches; he who abides in me and I in him, he bears much fruit, for apart from me, you can do nothing.

Abide? How does one do that? Abide means to remain or continue. So, continue following His teachings and examples and ways, as though He would always be with you. One of the Hebrew translations would have been to cleave, follow close, joined together as if glued. A vine is connected to the branch in a symbiotic relationship. Without the Branch, fruit cannot be born, for it is in the Branch the life blood flows. Continue in His Word daily. As you follow in His teachings, others will begin to see the fruit that is formed. The fruit of love, joy, peace, patience, kindness, goodness, faithfulness, gentleness and self- control. There is a flip side to this. What happens when we do not abide? Well then it becomes spiritual suicide. Those who are not Christ- followers do not understand this, for they do not know what it is to have an abundant life, filled with joy, amidst sorrow, and hardships. To abide is to continually confess to Jesus that I cannot live my life without Him. He knows that. He told His disciples that. He told me that and you and anyone else who would read His Word.

<u>Prayer</u>: Dear Father, who art in heaven, thank you that you are my heavenly Father and you tend to my life with such care and concern. Cleanse me and prune me, and take away anything that you discover in me that does not glorify your holy name. Thank you Father that you fill me with your fullness so that I may live and move and grow and bear fruit as I abide more and more in You each day. In Jesus name. Amen

DAY 3: Eat the Word of God

Scripture: Jeremiah 15vs16 your Words were found and I ate them, and your Words became for me a joy and the delight of my heart, for I have been called by your name, O Lord God of host.

The word of the Lord is pure and righteous altogether. The word of the Lord stands fast for ever and ever and we are exhorted to hear and preach the word- to obey and meditate on the word of God and to read and learn and inwardly digest its many truths. If we are to show ourselves approved unto God. We are called to be doers of the word and not hearers only- and we are to trust in its precepts and promises and not to despise or hold tightly the living word of truth. Jeremiah treasured up the word of God in his heart and it became his joy and delight and he readily received all that the Lord had to offer. In the same way as a hungry man devours a life sustaining meal. Then as now the word of the Lord is sweet and wholesome. It is nourishing, nutritious and strengthening and life-sustaining- for in it there is all we need for life and godliness. But the word of the Lord also contains some severe warnings, for both nations and individuals as well as many lovely promises. None of us are free from the difficulties and dangers of life, nor are we exempt from the correction hand of our God and His rod of discipline. In our life and on our world, as Jeremiah also discovered. Let us, like Jeremiah, continue to share the good news of the gospel of grace and warn others of the corrective hand of our God on our lives and our world. Let us be prepared to warn of His rod of discipline and fast approaching judgement of the nations, no matter what negative reactions we relieve from others- knowing that the Word of the Lord is pure and righteous altogether and stands fast for ever and ever.

Prayer: Heavenly Father, thank you for your written Word and for Jesus Christ, the living Word of God. I pray that Your Word would become for me a joy and the delight of my heart. For I have been called by your name and saved by the blood of the lamb. I pray that I may be a doer of the Word and always trust in its precepts and promises, no matter what difficulties and dangers I may have to undergo as an individual or nationally. Help me to hold fast that which is good and do only those things that are pleasing in your sight. In Jesus name I pray. Amen.

DAY 4: Bread Is Not Enough

<u>Scripture</u>: **Matthew 4 vs 4 Jesus answered, "It is written: Man shall not live on bread alone but on every word that comes from the mouth of God."**

The word of God is essential in the life of anyone who claims to be a follower of Christ. The Bible tells us how to become a Christian and then how to follow Jesus in our everyday living. The word of God was important in the life of Jesus. It sustained Him and helped Him in times of temptation. We need to understand that the word of God is our sustenance. We live by every word that comes from the mouth of God. It is the word of God that gives us the strength to face the realities and difficulties of life. Therefore we must pay careful attention to what the Lord is saying to us. We need to live by the word of God. The word of God gives stability to our lives. Jesus said that whoever listens to His words and obeys them is like a wise man who built his house on the rock. When we build our lives on the word of God, we can face any storm and still remain strong and stable. The word of God gives us security and an assurance of fulfillment. Jesus said that even if heaven and earth pass away, His words would never pass away. God is not a man that He should lie or change His mind. We can trust His promises with full assurance. He will fulfill what He has promised. The word of God rescues us from danger and destruction. The Lord sends His word in times of crisis and desperation and heals us and delivers us from the grave. The word of God will not return empty, but will accomplish what He desires and achieve the purpose for which He sent it. People need more than bread to live; we must feed on every word of God because it helps us in times of need and it transforms us and gives us the understanding and assurance of eternal life where we have " the right to eat from the tree of life, which is in the paradise of God. **What are you feeding on?**

<u>Prayer</u>: **Teacher God, thank you for your scripture. Jesus showed me that I should follow the Word just as He did. Teach me, remind me, and guide me to know the Word of God and live by it. I want to be a disciple for you. Amen.**

DAY 5: Grow in your Salvation

<u>Scripture:</u> **1 Peter 2vs 2 "Like newborn babies, crave pure spiritual milk, so that by it you may grow up in your salvation."**

Many think, once we accept Jesus as our Savior, we will just know what is true. However, if we are not studying God's Word and feeding spiritually on His truth, we are vulnerable to living more by what we feel than what is true, which over time is sure to lead us astray. Too often we don't realize if we don't know the Word of God, even when we are believers, we can be led astray. Knowing what scripture says helps us to discern if what we are hearing and reading is based on God's truth or on the enemy's lies. **1 Peter 2vs2** encourages, when it comes to the Word of God, we want to be like newborn babies who crave pure spiritual milk, so that we may grow up in our salvation. So what is this pure spiritual milk? God's Word is the milk needed in our progress to eating solid foods, which are the deeper truths. So why is it so important to grow spiritually as a Christian? Is it enough to just be saved? If we don't grow in our knowledge of God's word we become vulnerable to being deceived and led astray by the evil one. Unfortunately, so many Christians become discouraged, feeling like they cannot even read God's Word on their own, thinking they don't have the education or capability to understand it. However Jesus tells us, we can rely on the Holy Spirit to teach us all things.

<u>Prayer:</u> **Heavenly Father, thank you for your Word, which has all we need for life and godliness. Thank you for the lessons it teaches and for its cleansing power. May we sincerely desire the pure milk of the Word so that we may grow in grace, mature in the faith and become increasingly conformed into the image and likeness of the Lord Jesus, in whom name I pray. Amen**

DAY 6: God Always Provide

<u>Scripture:</u> **Genesis 1vs29 And God said, "Behold, I have given you every plant yielding seed that is on the face of all the earth, any every tree with seed in its fruit. You shall have them for food."**

We should always take heart that God will always provide for His children. God's desire is to provide for us by blessing us to work. But even when we work hard for our food, we should understand that the outcome of our hard work belongs to the Lord. Our hard work is even the Lord working through us. Everything we have is from God. We have nothing, no matter how hard we worked for it, that God has not provided. Whenever Jesus broke bread to eat, He gave thanks because He knew all that we have is given to us. God entrusted the stewardship of the whole earth to man, His delegated authority over creation. He has provided for our sustenance only those plants and fruits that are digestible for us. God knows what we need, and we can take Him at His Word. We, who are saved through faith in Christ are one part of that precious plan of salvation. We are members of the body of Christ, and we are positioned in Him.

<u>Prayer:</u> **Heavenly Father, thank you for the Word of God and the beautiful truth it contains. Thank you that despite man's sin, you placed in motion your perfect plan of redemption. Thank you for faith in Jesus, I am a new creation in Him and part of His spiritual body. May I live and work to your praise and glory, in Jesus name I pray. Amen.**

DAY 7: Great Invitation

<u>Scripture:</u> Isaiah 55 vs 1-2 "Come everyone who thirst, come to the waters; and he who has no money, come by and eat! Come, buy wine and milk without money and without price. Why do you spend your money for that which is not bread, and your labor for that which does not satisfy? Listen diligently to me.

Let me ask dear brothers and sisters in Christ: How do you feel about our task of sharing the gospel of Jesus Christ with others? Does the idea of proclaiming the Good News of Jesus to your unsaved friends, family members, neighbors and work associates excite you? Does it motivate you? Are you driven to do it? Do you earnestly pray for opportunities from God to point other people to Jesus? And when those opportunities come, do you grasp them with eagerness and enthusiasm and a genuine passion? To be honest, most of us don't greet such opportunities with anything like eagerness or enthusiasm or passion. Sometimes, we hesitate because we don't feel that evangelism is our particular "gift." All too often, we fail in our faith because we are too busy and distracted by things of this world. Sometimes we are silent because we are afraid of what might happen if we bear witness to Jesus that we might confuse people because we didn't share it correctly: or that we might raise the anger of people who are strong in their unbelief; or that we might disturb the peace of people around us. This devotion is not intended to be judge mental but to get us to become zealous about God himself and give others the privilege of sharing with them our Lord and Savior.

<u>Prayer:</u> Heavenly Father, forgive us as you have given us opportunities to minister to the lost but as a result, we said nothing for whatever reason. Help us- now- today to find fulfillment in your love and to share that love with others so that they also can be free to honor your name. Amen.

DAY 8: Being Truly Wise

Scripture: Proverbs 3vs 7-8 "Be not wise in your own eyes; fear the Lord and turn from evil. It will be healing to your flesh and refreshments to your bones."

We as humans have a tendency to overestimate ourselves and to think that we know better than anyone else. All of us have known people who refuse to be corrected under any circumstances, and all of us at times have refused to be corrected ourselves. These realities manifest our inclination to exalt our own "wisdom" above the wisdom of others, an inclination that goes right back to the beginning. The primal sin in Eden was the creature's false belief that he was wiser than the Creator. Adam and Eve chose to partake of the forbidden fruit because they chose to believe that they knew better than the Creator himself, that it was wiser to do what they wanted rather than obey the Lord's admonition not to eat of the tree of knowledge of good and evil. If unfallen creatures could give into that temptation and plunge the human race into ruins, how much more are we sinners not to trust in ourselves above all else? This scripture warns us not to be wise in our own eyes. We must trust first and foremost in the Lord and His Word, and secondly in the godly wisdom evident in the lives of those who serve Him faithfully. We are to trust the Lord with all our hearts and lean not on our own understanding by revealing the blessings. As scripture often does, today's passage encourages us to trust in the Lord by revealing the blessings that follow such trust--- "healing to our flesh and refreshment to our bones."

Prayer: Lord, I thank you that you are the God of the impossible. You can do anything. I want to trust in your ability and not my own. Teach me to see difficulties in my life from your perspective. Help me to focus and lean on you and your power. In Jesus name. Amen.

DAY 9: God Has Given Us Everything We Need

<u>Scripture:</u> 2 Peter 1vs3 By His divine power, God has given us everything we need for living a godly life. We have received all of this by coming to know Him; the one who called us to himself by means of his marvelous glory and excellence.

We ask God anxiously, "Give me this "as if God were withholding some good thing from us. But that is not the case at all. That's not what God is like at all! That kind of thinking dishonors God, because he's already given us everything we need. Isn't that a great reason for contentment, whatever may be our circumstances? Even more, it should lead us to continual gratitude and rejoicing. Peter goes on to tell us that we have access to what God has already given us that it is through these promises that we are able to escape the world's corruption. It's our desires that are the problem, because we want more, than what God has given us as if his gifts weren't good enough, as if we needed more. Our problem is that we fail to respond to God's promises. We think that Christian growth is based on our own efforts, rather than accepting and resting on the promises of God. He has already given us everything that we need!

<u>Prayer:</u> Heavenly Father, I humbly come before you with a grateful heart, praising you with all my being, for I know that every good perfect gift comes from you. The   one who never changes. As I lift up this prayer, I also recognize my forgetfulness in giving you thanks each and every day. May I learn to thank you daily for giving me everything that I need In Jesus' name Amen.

DAY 10: Live Overflowing

<u>Scripture:</u> **Ephesians 5vs18 Do not get drunk on wine, which leads to debauchery, Instead, be filled with the Spirit**
It is interesting that Paul puts these two things in contrast, one against the other. Don't get drunk with wine, he says. This recognizes that there are things in life that tend to drive you to drink. There are pressures in life and many demands made upon you so severe that you will feel the need of some stimulation, something that will undergird you a bit, give you some confidence and help and strength. "But don't let it be wine or any other artificial stimulant because he says, "the trouble with that is, it so easily leads to lack of control. " The word that means "without any limits, with reckless abandonment," it refers to escapism and the tendency to throw all restraints overboard and without control. But in contrast to that, he says to satisfy that need for something to stimulate and strengthen you by being filled with the Spirit, for that is God's provision for this need in human life. We were not made to be self-sufficient, independent creatures. Because you feel like you need something to help you, to strengthen you, to make you feel adequate to face life, do not be troubled by that. You do need something. But let it be the right thing. "Be filled with the Spirit." The great secret of real Christianity, the possibility of being filled with the Spirit. You have the Spirit, but the interesting paradox is that, though all Christians have the Holy Spirit, we constantly need to be filled with the Holy Spirit. How do you react to the severe demands and pressures of life? Are you learning to acknowledge the Spirit of Christ within and to be overflowing with His Presence?

<u>Prayer:</u> **Father, I pray that you will teach me to draw upon the well of water within, to know that every demand made upon me is a demand made upon you, and that you are prepared, ready, to live your life through me in every situation and this manifests your grace. In Jesus name. Amen.**

DAY 11: Stop Worrying!

<u>Scripture:</u> **Philippians 4vs6 do not worry about anything: instead, pray about everything. Tell God what you need, and thank him for all he has done.**

Worry takes away our joy, apart from making us miserable, it has a lot of negative health implications. The Bible encourages us to "Always be full of joy in the Lord." Instead of worrying about things, the Word of the Lord recommends that we pray about it and tell the Lord what we need." Not only that, we should also thank him for all He has done." The remedy for worry is prayer. When you find yourself in extremely challenging circumstances, the default response is to worry. I encourage you not to. Why not talk to God about it and thank Him for every other thing He has done for you in the past. This will give you the much needed peace. Worry does not resolve problems, prayer does! Worry is the opposite of faith. It steals our peace, physically wears us out, and can even make us sick. When we worry, we torment ourselves—we're doing the devil's job for him! Worry is caused by not trusting God to take care of the various situations in our lives. Too often we trust our own abilities, believing that we can figure out how to take care of our own problems. And yet, after all our worry and effort to go it alone, we come up short—unable to bring about suitable solutions. Too often our experiences in the world teach us this, and even after we become Christians, it takes a long time to overcome it. It's difficult to learn how to trust God, but we eventually must learn that trying to take care of everything ourselves, is too big a task.

<u>Prayer</u>: **Lord Jesus, I accept your word as the truth. Lord, I am worried about________. Instead of worrying, I ask that you help me find a solution to the problem. I also thank you for all you have done for me in the past. This I pray in Jesus' name. Amen!**

DAY 12: Supper Time

<u>Scripture:</u> I Corinthians 11vs23-25 For I received from the Lord what I also delivered to you, that the Lord Jesus on the night when He was betrayed took bread, and when He had given thanks, He broke it, and said, "This is my body, which is for you. Do this in remembrance of me. In the same way also He took the cup, after supper, saying, "This cup is the new covenant in my blood. Do this as often as you drink it, in remembrance of me.

The only sinners who can freely commune with Jesus at His table are those who have acknowledged that they are sinners and have turned to Him as their only hope in life and in death. Do not let feelings of unworthiness prevent you from coming to His table. Jesus invites you to come and sit with Him if you are following Him in a life of repentance and faith. The Lord is truly present every time we take the sacrament with other believers. As you take the supper, consider the presence of Christ and the way He meets all our needs. In celebrating the Lord's Supper we are given a special opportunity to reflect on the new creation that is coming and to set our hope on Christ, who will surely bring to completion all that He has started. Let us look forward to this glorious day whenever we eat the bread and drink the wine in the sacrament of the Lord of the Lord's Supper is that it spiritually feeds us with Christ Himself. As we partake of the Lord's Supper, we may come to His table for grace and strength. In the Lord's Supper we receive true nourishment of our souls. When was the last time you partaken in the Lord's Supper? What were your feelings afterwards?

<u>Prayer:</u> Father God, You have called me to be a person for your own self and so help me to unify in spirit and in purpose, to do the things you have appointed us to do, and this includes partaking and participating in the Lord's Supper as a body, which we are commanded to do. Since this is your body, the church, we know that you are present with us, and that you are in each and every one of us: you are our all and all. We give you glory for your amazing grace.

DAY 13: Appreciating Our Bodies

<u>Scripture:</u> 1 Corinthians 6vs19-20You are not your own; you were bought at a price. Therefore honor God with your bodies.

Scripture teaches us that our bodies are temples of the Holy Spirit. As Christians we are called to honor God with our bodies, and that includes valuing them and taking care of them. Remember that Jesus gave his own body to save us. Now we are encouraged to be good stewards of both body and soul, for we belong to God both physically and spiritually. This is another way to show our gratitude to God- by maintaining what He gave us through exercise and healthy eating habits. God wants us to be as healthy and fit as possible, as we serve him and our neighbor. Do you take good care of yourself and appreciate what Jesus did for you? If you don't take care of yourself, what good are you to anyone else? Self- Care and self- love are so important. Let's ask ourselves:
Can we do God's work at our best if we are feeling tired or sluggish?

Can we serve Him at our best if our minds are foggy because we haven't fueled our bodies with enough fuel? Taking care of our bodies is not about vanity! That's what the media wants us to believe. We take care of our bodies because it is in His word. We are to offer our body as a living sacrifice.   Our bodies are given to us to do His work. A healthy body gives us the energy to do God's work. As Christians taking caring of our bodies is taking care of the place where the Holy Spirit dwells.

<u>Prayer:</u> Lord I am thankful for the body of Jesus that was broken for us. Help us to grow in our appreciation of our own bodies as temples of the Holy Spirit. Amen.

DAY 14: Focus on Doing & Finishing the Work

<u>Scripture:</u> **John 4vs31-34 in the meantime, the disciples pressed him, "Rabbi, eat. Aren't you going to eat?" 'He told them "I have food to eat you know nothing about." The disciples were puzzled. Who could have brought him food? Jesus said "The food that keeps me going is that I do the will of the one who sent me, finishing the work he started."**

This is so profound when Jesus said "My nourishment comes from doing the will of God who sent me, and from finishing his work. "Jesus was talking about His life….But it hit me as I was studying this that He is also talking about ours! We live in a generation where even seasoned believers can be overwhelmed at how to find purpose in this media- driven ever-changing, confusing, loud and busy world! If we slow down long enough to think about it, though, that verse makes absolute sense for our lives and not just the life of Jesus. As a believer, when do you feel most deeply satisfied? Isn't it when you truly know you are making a difference that will last? Your example will last beyond your life. Your kindness, your meanness, your giving nature, your selfish stingy nature. Without trying…. We are making a difference not just for today or this week or a few years. We are making a difference for generations. Our children, nephews and nieces, friends ' children are focused by the most simple of actions. You don't always have to preach a sermon with your words but if you want to help finish the work that Jesus started, then you need to never stop or give up during the journey. The bonus is not only with the ones you influence but nourish also. What is God's will for you? What is it that nourishes you?

<u>Prayer:</u> **Dear Jesus, help me to focus on those things you have a purpose for me to complete. The task that you have set out for me to accomplish. I thank you that I have your mind, I know your will. Help me to obey your leading to be sensitive to your promptings. May I finish the race set before me well! Amen.**

DAY 15: Turning Point

<u>Scripture:</u> John 6vs 63-64 Jesus said "The Spirit gives life; the flesh counts for nothing. The word I have spoken to you--- they are full of the Spirit and life. Yet there are some of you who do not believe."

It was a turning point in Christ's ministry. For a while, many people followed Him because they expected Jesus to fulfill their own longings for the nation, people and personal lives. Christ's mission, however, was about fulfilling what God wanted, which ultimately meant some people would not do what they expected. Christ was adamant about what He was sent to do. His ministry had grown beyond their expectations, Jesus had come to bring salvation to the entire world. In a society that is obsessed with our physical well- being to the exclusion of our spiritual growth, what Jesus said is still difficult to accept. We spend so much of our earthling time and resources trying to keep our bodies healthy and pure that we tend to forget two things: 1.We are not physically immortal and 2. Our spirits are eternal. In the end it's not how we physically appear that is going to be important. So perhaps next time we look at starting a new diet plan or an exercise regime, we should also set aside the same amount of time, energy and effort to go to church, read the Bible, and pray daily to God. After all, as Jesus said "The Spirit gives life: the flesh counts for nothing." Ask yourself: Am I as focused on holiness as I am on healthiness?

<u>Prayer:</u> Lord Jesus, encourage us to look after our spirits and grow in faith. Enable us to accept each day as an opportunity to grow closer to you. In Your Holy name, I pray. Amen.

DAY 16: You Are Bless!

<u>Scripture:</u> **Matthew 5vs6 blessed are those who hunger and thirst for righteousness for they will be filled.**

In this verse Jesus is describing the heart of a person who is sold out to God. He uses the words "hunger and thirst" to describe an un-quenching desire for the righteousness of God. Of course the righteousness of God that is being referenced here refers to all the Spiritual blessings that come when one is found in right standing with God. When we are standing in Christ righteousness, the Holy Spirit will develop within us a strong desire for the righteousness of God and all that it entails. Through the process of sanctification, God will begin to reshape our hearts. The promise is that those who hunger and thirst for righteousness "will be filled." Those who sincerely desire Spiritual blessings are blessed in those desires and shall be filled with those blessings. It is a desire of God's own raising, and He will not forsake the work of His own hands. Our soul is going to hunger and thirst after something. This is part of our Spiritual DNA. It is only God who can fill a soul, whose grace and favor are more than adequate to quench our deepest desires. He will fill those, who, with a sense of their own emptiness, have recourse to His fullness. What are your deepest desires? Do you find yourself gravitating toward the world and that it has to offer? How are you experiencing the blessings of peace and security that come from knowing that you are in right-standing with God?

<u>Prayer:</u> **Father, Your ways are higher than my ways. God, I want to live with the perspective of eternity. Set my eyes and heart on you. Please give me a holy hunger and thirst as only you can do. I pray that I will be filled. I pray this in Jesus' name. Amen.**

DAY 17: Where Is Your Fruit?

Scripture: Luke 6vs44 each tree is recognized by its own fruit. People do not pick figs from thorn bushes, or grapes from briers.

In Luke 6 Jesus is not just talking about trees, He is talking about people. People can be known by what they produce. On the outside, everything can look good, but the fruit that is produced might not be as pleasant as the outward appearance. Faith has a way of producing fruit in us. Faithful prayer and a community of believers around us cannot help produce the fruit of justice, peace, good news, grace, love and forgiveness. Good trees bear good fruit and bad trees bear bad fruit. Jesus' words here are a powerful warning that there are many who come in His name who are actually seeking to lead us away from the faith and we are to be on guard against this threat. We as sheep must always be alert and ready for such predators. And if the wolves can dress up a sheep, the threat becomes infinitely more severe. Jesus chose very strong words here to emphasize our need to be ever vigilant against a subtle but hostile threat to us and our brothers and sisters in Christ. What kind of fruit is faith producing in you? If the product of your life isn't very good, it is time to take a look at the tree of your life.

Prayer: Father please help me to examine the fruit of our lives. Fill me with faith that is strong from the roots up so that my fruit will be good and pleasing to you. Amen.

DAY 18: Bring the Flavor

Scripture: Matthew 5vs13 you are the salt of the earth. But if the salt loses its saltiness, how can it be made salty again? It is no longer good for anything, except to be thrown out and trampled underfoot by men.

Salt has two purposes first, to preserve food which would quickly spoil in the desert environment. Believers in Christ are preservatives to the world, preserving it from the evil inherent in the society of ungodly men whose unredeemed nature are corrupted by sin. Secondly, salt was used then, as now, as a flavor enhancer. In the same way that salt enhances the flavor of the food it seasons, the followers of Christ stand out as those who "enhance" the flavor of life in this world. Christians, living under the guidance of the Holy Spirit and obedience to Christ, will inevitably influence the world for good, as salt has a positive influence on the flavor of the food it seasons. Where there is strife we are to be peacemakers, where there is sorrow, we are to be ministers of Christ, binding up wounds and where there is hatred, we are to exemplify the love of God in Christ, returning good for evil. What are you seasoning?

Prayer: Father I pray that I will not lose my saltiness but will bring back the flavor to a bland world. Jesus, allow my faith to flavor everything I do and say every day. In Jesus name. Amen

DAY 19: Do Not Give God Your Scraps

<u>Scripture:</u> **Malachi 1 vs 8 Try offering then to your governor! Would he be pleased with you? Would he accept you? Says the Lord almighty.**

God is our greatest authority. We wouldn't give our earthly authorities our scraps. Yet so often we offer God the leftover portions of our time, money, energy, thought, and emotions. He gets the scraps and rejects--- just as the Israelites were offering the worst of their animals in sacrifice. We face a similar temptation. We pray with the five extra minutes we might have and aren't sure what else we can do with that time. We are happy givers' as long as we have some disposable income. We have to admit though, that extras are not really sacrifices. When we willingly sacrifice time, money, or energy that have value to us, it settles the greater value of God into our hearts and minds. God sacrificed His only Son for us. Certainly He is far more worthy of our best than any earthly authority. Applying to ourselves, let us remember what the Lord commands us to offer. Paul says, in His name, present your bodies as living sacrifice. We are to serve in the newness of the spirit. Sacrificing our bodies is not only keeping its members in all purity, as we would be members of Christ body, but also giving to the Lord that from which all purity must come, a heart devoted to His service and well instructed for that purpose in all heavenly knowledge and spiritual wisdom. Are you giving your best?

<u>Prayer:</u> **Dear Jesus, please forgive me for not treating you according to your full value. I want you to have my best. I want you to have my extras too. I want to be fully yours. Amen.**

DAY 20: Refreshing Shepard

<u>Scripture:</u> Psalms 23:2-3 He makes me lie down in green pastures, He leads me beside quiet waters, he refreshes my soul.

Psalms 23 declares that the Lord is my Shepherd and the shepherd desire is to refresh my soul. There are two powerful blessings in this refreshing. First, the shepherd knows that life beats our soul. Life is often confusing, we have to make all kinds of decisions. We try to love people and mess up at times. We make plans and they often fall apart. Every day we deal with situations that may have us feeling anxious, weary, and discouraged. Our souls need constant refreshing, and the shepherd knows this so well therefore He walks right alongside us. Secondly, the shepherd knows we need green pastures and quiet waters. The beauty here is that these pastures and waters can be different for all of us! Your green pastures and quiet waters may be different from mine. But the shepherd knows you better than you know yourself and He will lead you to the right places for refreshment. When we surrender to His leading, God takes me places where weary exhaustion begins to die and life is refreshed. Are you being refreshed daily? Do you feel dried out? Overworked? If so, commit these concerns to the Lord.

<u>Prayer:</u> Shepherd of life, help me see the green pastures and quiet waters you are leading me to, and restore my soul. In Jesus name. Amen!

DAY 21: Breakfast with Jesus

<u>Scripture:</u> John 21:12 Jesus said to them, "Come and have breakfast." Now, none of the disciples dare ask Him. "Who are you?" They knew it was the Lord.

Have you made a mistake in the past that continues to stand out as a painful memory? Does that event continue to define you? What does God think of your past offenses? Let's look at Peter who failed miserably by denying that he even knew his friend Jesus. The event was marked by a rooster crowing. Jesus looking at Peter and Peter weeping bitter tears of remorse. Now Peter and Jesus meet again. How will Jesus treat someone who abandoned him in his darkest hour? Will Jesus be angry and want to punish Peter? Does Jesus ignore him? No. As the disciples were fishing, they saw Jesus on the shore. He called out to them saying "Friends, haven't you caught any fish? "No", they answered. He said "Throw your net on the right side of the boat and you will remain faithful and bless them with a miraculous catch of fish. Then, Jesus invites them to 'come and have breakfast. Such a warm gesture of friendship and hospitality. Next comes the crucial part of the story: Jesus addresses Peter's denial by asking him three times. "Do you love me? Jesus does not ignore the past; He addresses it. And the denials are cancelled out by Peter's new statements of love for Jesus. Regardless of what you have done in the past, Jesus calls you to come and follow Him too. Will you come, so you too can be forgiven?

<u>Prayer:</u> Jesus, I want to come. Accept and love me. Help me to realize that whatever I have done in the past you continue to welcome me with loving arms and forgiveness. I pray in Jesus' name. Amen.

BONUS SECTION
Daily Affirmation with Scriptures

<u>Scripture:</u> Proverbs 18vs21 states that "The tongue has the power of life and death, and those who love it will eat its fruit.

I decided to add this bonus section because I realize that the way you see things determine how you view your life. I wanted to inform you that you have the power to change the direction of your life no matter how it looks. Our words have a creative power. Whenever we speak something either positive or negative, we give life to what we are saying. We do this not realizing that we are prophesying our own futures. The scripture says, "We will eat its fruit." Meaning we will get exactly what we have been saying. You cannot speak defeat and expect victory. You cannot speak what you do not have and expect to receive an abundance of blessings. What are you speaking over yourself and others? Here is a list of powerful affirmations you can speak over yourself and others.

I don't worry about everyday life. God knows my needs and meets them because I make His Kingdom my primary concern. Matthew 6:25-33

Jesus shows himself to me because I love him. John 14:21

Because Jesus died for my sins, I am no longer separated from God. I live in close union with him. Romans 5:10

I can see the Kingdom of God because I am born again. John 3:3

The fruit I produce brings great joy to God, my Father in Heaven. John 15:8

God's power works best in my weakness. 2 Corinthians 12:9

Through the energy of Christ working powerfully in me, I teach others His truths. Colossians 1:29

I have been saved, not by works, but grace, so that I might do good works. Ephesians 2:9-10

My faith makes me whole in spirit, soul and body. Mark 5:34

When I call out to God He answers me. He tells me things I wouldn't know otherwise. Jeremiah 33:3

Because I place my hope in the Lord my strength is renewed. Isaiah 40:31

As I follow Jesus.....as I walk with him, I have peace. Luke 24:36

Because I obey Jesus I remain in his love. John 15:10

The cross of Christ is my power. 1 Corinthians 1:17

My God meets all my needs. Philippians 4:19

God is my refuge and strength …. always ready to help me in times of trouble. Psalm 46:1

God gives me strength when I am weary and increases my power when I am weak. Isaiah 40:29

Because I place my hope in God, I can soar like an eagle, run and not grow weary, walk and not be faint. Isaiah 40:31

I set my heart and mind on things above, not earthly things. This gives me peace. Colossians 3:1-2

I guard my heart because it determines the course of my life. Proverbs 4:23

I trust God at all times because he is my refuge. Psalm 62:8

As I lose my life for Jesus' sake, I find it. Matthew 10:39

God keeps me in perfect peace because I trust in Him and fix my thoughts on Him. Isaiah 26:3

God is able to do immeasurably more in my life than I could ever imagine. Ephesians 3:20

I experience true life when I deny myself, turn from my selfish ways and follow Jesus. Matthew 16:24-25

I have the anointing of Jesus, through the Holy Spirit. He teaches me truth and empowers me to live a full life. 1 John 2:27

I love God's principles and meditate on them all day long. Psalm 119:97

I live by faith, not by sight. 2 Corinthians 12:7

I follow Jesus, no matter where he leads me. Matthew 6:20

The same love that God has for Jesus is in me. John 17:26

I am being made holy by God's truths. John 17:17

It is by the grace of God and his love that I am saved by my faith. Ephesians 2:5

I can approach God directly with freedom and confidence through faith in Jesus. Ephesians 3:12

I worship the Lord my God and serve only him. Luke 4:8

I have great joy because I obey God's commands and remain in His love! John 15:11

Because I have written love and faithfulness on the tablet of my heart I have favor with God. Proverbs 3:3

The "fullness of God" is available to me because I am deeply rooted in the love of Jesus. Ephesians 3:17-19

As I give up control, release my life 2 God and allow Jesus to live through me, God-sized things happen. Galatians 2:20

I do not live by bread alone, but by every word that proceeds from the mouth of God. Matthew 4:4

Because I believe in God and in Jesus, trouble leaves my heart. John 14:1

God pours out his love into my heart by the Holy Spirit. Romans 5:5

My life is bringing honor to Christ. God likes this. Philippians 1:20

Because I fear the Lord and shun evil, my body is healthy and my bones are nourished. Proverbs 3:7-8

As I follow Jesus and walk in his Way of Holiness, gladness and joy overtake me. Isaiah 35:8-10

The Lord is my good Shepherd. He provides for all of my needs. Psalm 23:1

I was made in the image of God. How cool is that! Genesis 1:27

God reveals his spiritual truths to me by his Holy Spirit. 1 Corinthians 2:13

In God I live and move and exist. Acts 17:28

I may never win an Olympic medal, but I've won a crown of everlasting joy because I know Christ. Isaiah 51:11

I continue to work out my full salvation as God works in me according to his good purpose. Philippians 2:12-13

God does not look at my outward appearance. He looks at my heart. 1 Samuel 16:7

Because I seek the Lord with all my heart, I lack no good thing Psalm 34:10

The key to my fruit-bearing life is hearing God's truth and understanding it. Matthew 13:23

When I humble myself before God in prayer, he hears me and I gain understanding. Daniel 10:12

My faith, that saves and transforms me, comes by reading and understanding God's Word. Romans 10:12

God's Holy Spirit, who lives in me, opens my mind to the deep truths in God's Word. 1 John 2:27

I'm like a tree, planted by streams of water. My life bears fruit and prospers because I meditate on God's Word. Psalm 1:1-2

More than anything else I try to guard my heart because it determines how I live life. Proverbs 4:23

I don't act thoughtlessly, but try to understand what the Lord wants me 2 do. Ephesians 5:17

God's Spirit in me is greater than any other spirit in the world. He enables me to live a victorious life. 1 John 4:4

I am experiencing real Life – as Jesus intended. 1 John 5:12

The Holy Spirit helps me understand God's truth when I read the Bible. John 16:12

Experiencing God and his truths, not knowledge about him and them, gives me abundant LIFE. John 17:3

Because I feed on bread that comes from heaven (Jesus) I have life.... and will live eternally. John 6:57-58

I give thanks to God because he is good and his love endures forever. Jeremiah 33:11

I don't hide my light under a basket. I let it shine for all to see so everyone will praise my Father. Matthew 5:15-16

God forgives my wrongdoings and never remembers my sins. Hebrews 8:12

I am a new person, complete in Christ. 2 Corinthians 5:17

If I don't stand firmly in my faith, I won't stand at all. Isaiah 7:9

I am able to keep my ways pure, but only by living according to God's Word. Psalm 119:9

I run along the paths of God's commands because He has set my heart free. Psalm 119:32

God is faithful. He'll complete the good work that he has begun in me. Philippians 1:6

I alone am not competent. My competence comes from God. 2 Corinthians 3:5

I give my anxieties to God and know that he'll take them because he loves me. This gives me peace. 1 Peter 5:7

The Lord stands at my side and gives me strength to share his Good News with others. 2 Timothy 4:17

As I lose my life for Christ's sake, I find true life in him. Matthew 10:39

I have life, now & eternally, because of God's grace. It's not because of anything I have done. Eph 2:8-9

Because I've walked through Jesus' gate, I've found green pastures. John 10:9

When I'm distressed, I cry to God for help and he hears my voice. Psalm 18:6

God quiets my deep inner hunger because I am cherished by him. Psalm 17:14

When I cry to God for relief from the deepest pits of my life, he hears me. Lamentations 3:55-56

When I'm distressed, I cry to God 4 help and he hears my voice. Psalm 18:6

If I don't stand firmly in my faith, I won't stand at all. Isaiah 7:9

God is love and he is in me, so I am love. 1 John 4:16

Thank you Jesus for counting me faithful and putting me into ministry.
1 Timothy 1:12

Jesus died and rose from the grave for me. I'm blessed because I believe this and have not seen him. John 20:29

Though I have not seen the resurrected Christ, I believe in Him and am therefore blessed. John 20:29

I am protected by the name of Jesus. John 17:12

The Lord is good! I've experienced him. Psalm 34:8

I have a living hope through the resurrection of Jesus from the dead. 1 Peter 1:3

Because of what Christ did on the cross at Calvary, I'm able to have a new life. John 10:10

When Christ died I was set free from the power of sin. Romans 6:6

My negative feelings don't come from God so I don't have to put up with them! 2 Timothy 1:7

Because God's Spirit lives in me, my spirit is alive and I have true life. Romans 8:11

Some day I'll be in heaven with my Father because I know the way there – Jesus! John 14:6

Jesus Christ gives me victory over sin and death. 1 Corinthians 15:57

When Jesus knocks on my heart's door I hear him, let him in and have fellowship with him. Revelation 3:20

Because I follow Jesus, I know his voice and he personally directs my steps. John 10:3

I do not fear death because it's my doorway to heaven. 1 Corinthians 15:55

The power of God works through me as I affirm that it's His treasure inside this jar of clay. 2 Corinthians 4:7

As I cast my cares and burdens to God, He sustains me and I have peace. Psalm 55:22

I am not afraid or discouraged because God goes before me and is always with me. Deuteronomy 31:8

I have entered the kingdom of God like a little child. Mark 10:15

My kind words are sweet to the soul and healing to the bones of others. Proverbs 16:24

God blesses me with peace and gives me strength. Psalm 29:11

As I wait on the Lord and am courageous, God will strengthen my heart. Psalm 27:14

My God is compassionate and merciful – slow to get angry and filled with unfailing love. Psalm 103:8

I try to spend time with wise people. This helps me become even wiser. Proverbs 13:20

I know the scripture, yes, but more importantly I know Jesus, and in Him I have life. John 5:39-40

CONCLUSION

God's Words are good for us to eat; we need to eat the Word of God daily. According to divine revelation in the Bible, the word of God is not only for us to understand and remember, but all the more for us to eat and digest. God's words are good for us to eat and we need to take that part of our Christian walk very seriously. God's word is the divine supply of food that nourishes us, and as we pray over the word of God, He dispenses His riches into our inner being to nourish us so that we may be constituted with the elements. The secret is that the word is Spirit and life to us; therefore, we need to exercise our spirit to pray over God's word. Receiving the word by means of prayer and we will be inwardly nourished with the divine supply of God's word. We need to learn how to pray and read the word so that we may eat and grow in life so that we can be a part of His corporate expression. Remember eating is a personal matter. I can't eat for you and you cannot eat for me. I pray that you have enjoyed this full- course meal that was delivered to you in this book of S.E.C.R.E.T.S.

Closing Prayer

Lord Jesus, I want to not be rebellious but come to you, eat the word of God, digest it, assimilate it, and speak the word of God which has been constituted into my being! Save me from merely sharing something that inspired me or touched me in your word. May I take the way of eating the word of God, devouring it, digesting it, and assimilating it, so that the word would operate in my being and become my very constitution. I want to eat the word of God without any kind of discrimination!

Lord I want to be those who find Your Word, eat them, and digest them, so that your word would become to me the gladness and joy of my heart. Thank you Lord that your Word is not merely for knowledge but for me to eat and be inwardly supplied! May I not be satisfied with merely reading the Bible, but may I dig deeper into God's word by praying over the word of God so that I may be inwardly supplied and nourished with the bountiful supply of the Spirit and the riches of Christ in Jesus name I pray. Amen. Amen & Amen.

www.ingramcontent.com/pod-product-compliance
Lightning Source LLC
Chambersburg PA
CBHW031435250726
48656CB00002B/993